FAC

Written by Chris Madsen
Illustrated by Cecelia Fitzsimmons and Lesley Smith

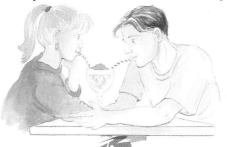

HENDERSON
PUBLISHING PLC

INTRODUCTION

WHY? WHY? WHY?

Have you ever asked somebody a question and got an answer which doesn't tell you what you really wanted to know? Have you ever asked two different people the same question and got two different answers? If this seems puzzling, it probably means that the question you asked was a very big one.

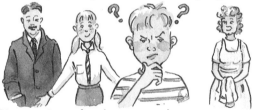

Big questions often have more than one answer, and asking 'why?' could get you any one of them. If you ask a lot of different people the same big question, and collect up all the different answers they give you, you'll end up with a good, big answer to a big question.

You probably want to ask a lot of questions about babies, and sex, and all the other things that come into your head once you start thinking about these things. You'll find a lot of the answers in this book, although they may not be in the first place you look.

Some questions may not interest you right now, so skip these until you feel like asking. Some questions might not have the exact answers you are looking for, but maybe you can use the answers you do find to help you work out a better question.

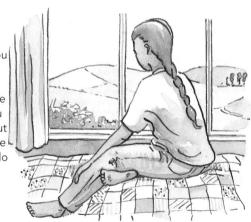

WHY AM I DIFFERENT?

Everyone is different. Every single person in the world is special. Nobody is exactly like anybody else who has ever lived, or will ever live in the future. Strange as it may seem, the reason for this is because we have two sexes, male and female. Because of sex, every time a new baby is made, a man and a woman each put part of their own special self into this new person, so that it is a brand-new combination of both of them.

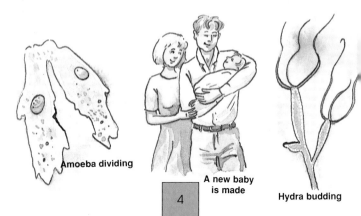

Amoeba dividing

A new baby
is made

Hydra budding

4

MAKING CHANGES

If anybody could make a new person, all alone, by simply splitting in two, which some animals and many plants can do, then we'd only be able to make lots more people who were exactly the same, over and over again. This would be very boring, but it would also mean that we would never be able to change, or evolve, because the main way that living things change is by sexual reproduction. If nature hadn't invented sex, we might not even exist!

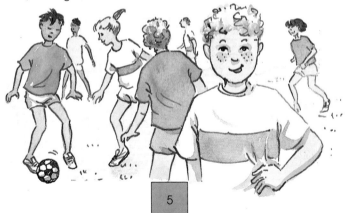

WHAT MAKES ME THE WAY I AM?

Each person's body contains a special set of instructions, written in a secret code called the genetic code. There's a copy of your own code in every tiny cell of your body. The code is quite simple, but the instructions make a very, very long list. They tell your body exactly how to make every bit of itself so, all the time you're growing, you're making more of your own special self.

There are instructions for the colour of your hair, for whether your hair will grow straight or curly, for whether you have fine or heavy hair, for how thickly your hair grows on your head, and for the thousands of other things that make you a special person.

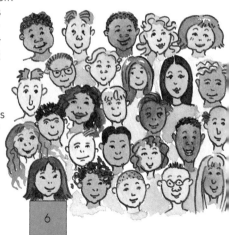

GENES AND CHROMOSOMES

The code message for each different thing is called a gene. One gene decides the colour of your hair, but another one will decide whether it is straight or curly. Altogether, everyone has around a hundred thousand different genes. Genes are joined up into long chains called chromosomes. There are 46 chromosomes, arranged into 23 pairs. Everybody has one of each pair, and each pair looks different.

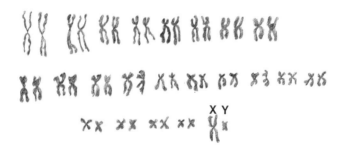

X Y

WHY DO I LOOK LIKE MY FAMILY?

Every new baby gets half of its code (23 chromosomes) from its mother, in the egg, and the other half (the other 23) from its father, in the sperm which fertilised the egg. You got your code from your own parents, which is why you look like them. Brothers and sisters have the same father and mother. Their chromosomes all come from the same two sets, so they could look a little or a lot like each other as well as looking like their parents.

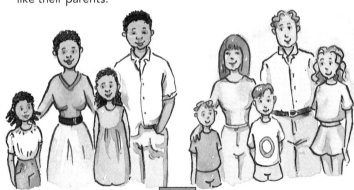

WHY AREN'T WE IDENTICAL?

The differences between brothers and sisters are caused because chromosomes get shuffled around when babies are made, something like the way a pack of cards is shuffled between games. The way it happens is a bit more interesting than this, but you can see how brothers and sisters can each be dealt a different hand even though the cards come from the same two packs. This means that it's almost impossible for two brothers or two sisters to get exactly the same code, except for identical twins.

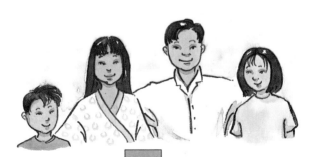

HOW DO TWINS HAPPEN?

Identical twins are completely different from fraternal (not identical) twins. Identical twins come from one egg, fertilised by one sperm. Long before they were born, the tiny egg they grew from split up into two halves. Each half then grew into a whole new baby. Identical twins are two babies from the very same egg, and have the very same genetic code.

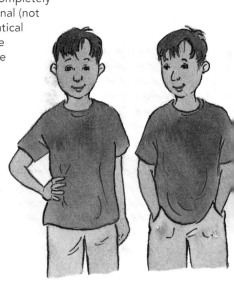

This is why they are always the same sex, and look so much alike. Sometimes it can be hard for their friends to tell them apart. This can make identical twins very unhappy, and it's important for their friends to understand that, even though they look alike, each one is a separate and special person.

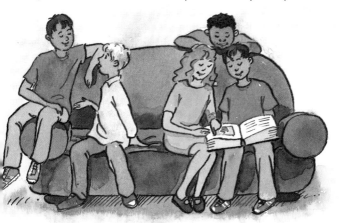

WHAT ABOUT OTHER TWINS?

Fraternal twins also grow inside their mother's womb at the same time, and are born on the same day. But they sometimes look very different from one another, and aren't always the same sex. Fraternal twins don't come from the same egg. They happen when two eggs were each fertilised and started to grow at the same time. Each egg has a different genetic code, so fraternal twins are like ordinary brothers or sisters except that they are both the same age.

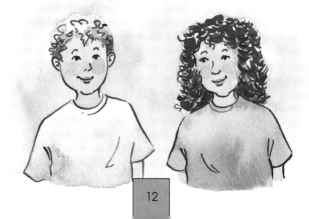

WHAT ARE SIAMESE TWINS?

Siamese twins get their name from the first famous pair, two boys named Chang and Eng, who were born in the country called Siam (which is now called Thailand). Chang and Eng were joined together at the chest, and they grew up and lived their whole lives this way.

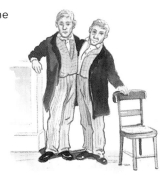

They both got married, and fathered 22 children altogether who were all perfectly normal. Nowadays, of course, Siamese twins joined in this way would be able to have an operation to separate them. Sometimes, though, a pair of Siamese twins are much more closely joined together. They might not even have two sets of all their body parts, and when this happens it may be impossible to save the lives of both babies.

HOW DO SIAMESE TWINS HAPPEN?

Quite simply, they are very unusual identical twins. When a single egg splits to make identical twins, the two halves nearly always come apart and grow quite separately. Very, very rarely, though, the two halves somehow stay stuck together, and then the two babies are still stuck together when they're born.

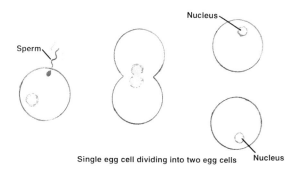

Nucleus

Sperm

Nucleus

Single egg cell dividing into two egg cells

DO TWINS RUN IN FAMILIES?

We know that fraternal twins do run in families, because some families have more than their fair share of these twins and others don't have any at all.

But nobody knows just what makes one egg split in half to make identical twins. Identical twins don't run in families, so any mother can suddenly find she's having two babies instead of just one.

Triplets are three babies who are born at the same time, and quads are four babies with the same birthday. Sometimes two of the triplets or quads are also identical twins. Can you work out why?

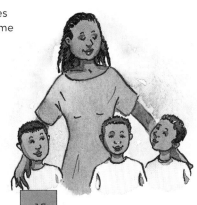

BOY OR GIRL – WHAT DECIDES?

Where did you get your own code, your own set of chromosomes from? You got them from your parents. Half of your 46 chromosomes came from your father, and the other half came from your mother. This is why they are arranged in pairs. Remember, too, that one of each pair is from your father and the other one is from your mother.

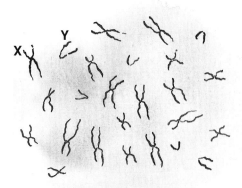

One pair of chromosomes isn't always a perfect match. A woman has a matching pair, but a man has a pair that look different. The woman's pair is called XX, because they look like two little Xs, and the man's pair is called XY, because that's what they look like.

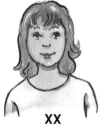

XX   **XY**

Your father's X came from his mother (your grandmother), and his Y came from his father (your grandfather). If you are a boy, you will have an X from your mother and a Y from your father. But if you're a girl, you will have got one X from your mother (who has two of them) and the other X from your father (who has one).

IT'S QUITE SIMPLE...

Each time two parents make a new baby, the baby gets half of all its chromosomes from its mother, and half from its father. If the baby gets its father's X (which gives it an X from both parents), it will be a girl. If it gets its father's Y chromosome, it will be a boy with an XY pair, like its father.

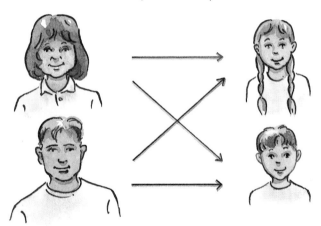

DO OUR GENES DECIDE EVERYTHING?

Even identical twins grow up to be different from one another. They never look exactly alike, and may enjoy doing different things.

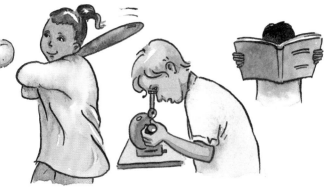

This is because, even though they have the very same genes, their bodies and their lives are also shaped by what happens to them after they are born.

IT'S UP TO US

The same is true for every one of us. What we're given to start with is only the beginning. We can't change things like the natural colour of our hair or the way it grows, but we can decide what hairstyle we want. The shape of our body can't be completely changed from the pattern which came from our own genetic code, but what we eat and how we use our body can make a big difference to the way it works and how it looks.

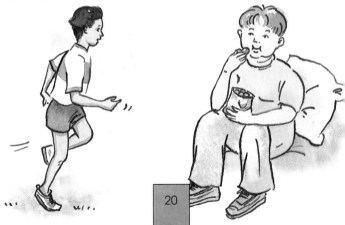

Some people have a special talent, but even this is only a start. We all have to work and practise the things we want to be good at, even if we are specially talented. Runners start by being able to run faster than their friends at school, but if they want to win Olympic gold medals they must decide to work and train very hard. Even our brain needs exercise, to help it work better.

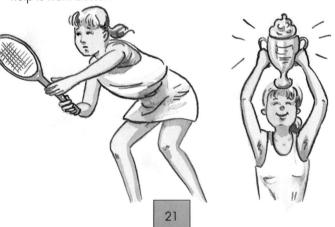

MAKE THE CHANGE

Everything else that happens to us can change the way we are, too. Sometimes the things that happen are good, and sometimes they aren't so good. But whatever we start out with, and whatever happens to us, each of us is a very special person, and each person can help himself or herself to become stronger, or healthier, or cleverer, or even happier.

When we are very young, our parents and our teachers make many decisions for us, but as we grow older we can gradually begin to make our own choices. By the time we are grown-up, we will be able to decide for ourselves what we want to do and what sort of person we'd like to be.

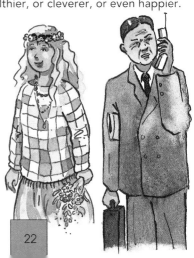

22

WHAT IS A MUTATION?

Once in a while, a baby is born who looks completely different from everyone else in the family. One reason why this can happen is because a gene in an egg or a sperm can suddenly change. Sudden changes in genes are called mutations. When a gene mutates, it can change the meaning of the whole code.

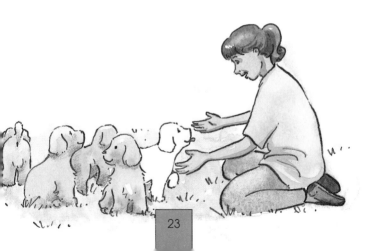

Usually, a big change like this makes the code into nonsense, in just the same way as a change in a single letter on this page could turn a whole sentence into nonsense. Most mutations spoil the genetic code so badly that it can't make a proper baby at all, and then no baby is born. Very, very rarely, though, a mutation happens which changes the code to give a new, sensible message. Then the result is a different, special baby. The new, changed gene might even be better than the old one, and this would make the new baby very special indeed.

WHAT MAKES MUTATIONS HAPPEN?

Mutations can happen all by themselves, but some things seem to make them happen more easily.

Two of the things which help mutations to happen are radioactivity and X-rays. The more radioactivity or X-rays a person's body collects, during their whole life, the bigger the chance of their eggs or sperms getting mutated (changed) genes in them.

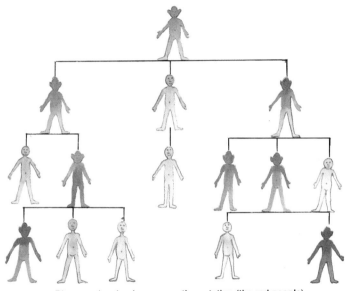

Diagram showing how a genetic mutation (the red people)
affects different generations

Because mutations are nearly always bad, we try to protect our genes by taking care not to get too much radioactivity or too many X-rays. It's quite safe to go to hospital to have an X-ray picture taken, but the person who works there (the radiographer) has to be in the same room with the X-ray machine every day, and so he or she takes care to hide behind a screen made of lead when the machine is working.

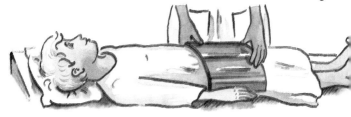

Lead is a very heavy metal which X-rays can't get through. Sometimes, when we go to have an X-ray, the radiographer gives us a heavy lead apron to wear. This prevents the X-rays from going near our eggs or sperms so it keeps their genes safe from mutating.

WHY DO GIRLS AND BOYS LOOK DIFFERENT?

A girl will grow up to be a woman, whose body makes eggs and then shelters and protects a growing baby until it is ready to be born.

A boy will grow up to be a man, whose body makes sperms.

Before a baby can start to grow, the egg which a woman makes must be fertilised by a sperm from a man. The egg is fertilised when a man's sperm and a woman's egg meet and join together.

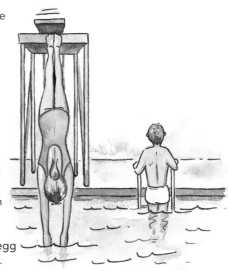

BACK TO BASICS

The egg and the sperm must meet inside a woman's body, where everything is just right for the baby to begin growing.

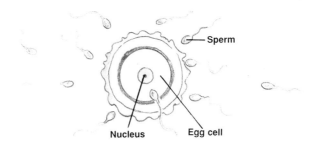

Sperm

Nucleus

Egg cell

So that this can happen, a man has to put his sperm right into a woman's body. This is why a man has a penis and a woman has an opening (called her vagina) between her legs.

When a man and a woman want to make a baby together, the man fits his penis into the woman's vagina to put the sperms right inside.

Although this won't happen until after they are grown up, these parts of boys' and girls' bodies are shaped differently from the start, ready for when they will be needed. The opening at the end of a man's penis is very small, so that it is hard for germs to get in. A woman's vagina has to be big enough to allow a penis inside and, later, to let a baby come out. To cover her vagina and protect it from germs, a woman has two folds of skin, called labia, which meet together in the middle.

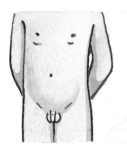 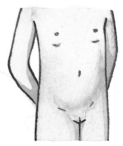

WHY DO BOYS AND GIRLS GO TO THE

Even when they're grown up, people don't spend very much of their time making babies or making love. Our bodies are built so that parts which aren't needed for one special thing all the time can do more than one thing. This is why we sometimes use our mouths to eat, sometimes to talk, sometimes to whistle, and sometimes to kiss.

Boys also use their penis for urinating (passing water; peeing), and because it's shaped like a short pipe this allows them to stand up and aim the urine where they want it to go.

Girls have to sit down to urinate because the urine simply flows from a small hole in front of their vagina and they can't choose which way it goes.

Both boys and girls sit down when they go to the lavatory to pass solids (faeces) from a different hole called the anus, which has its opening further back.

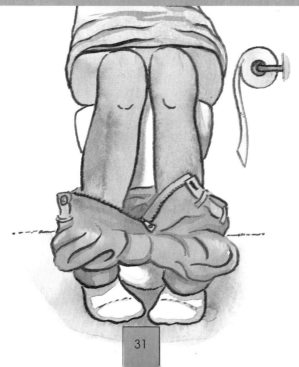

WHAT'S SPECIAL ABOUT A GIRL'S BODY?

The special part of a girl's body that is on the outside is called her vulva. Two pairs of skin-folds between her legs cover a moist, delicate place where there are two holes. The smaller hole in front, called the urethra, is for passing urine. The larger hole just behind it, called the vagina, will be used, one day when the girl is a woman, for letting in sperms and letting out babies. Until then, it is partly sealed with a thin skin called the hymen.

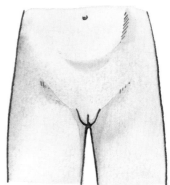

At the very front of the vulva, there is a small lump which is very ticklish. When a girl grows up, this ticklish lump, which is called the clitoris, will play an important part in making love. This is the part of a girl's body which is most like a boy's penis. It can swell, as a penis can, and become even more sensitive.

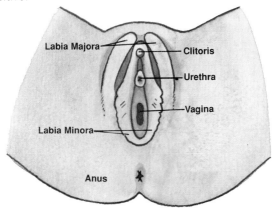

Inside, a girl's body also has a group of special parts. In the middle of the group is a small, hollow place where, one day when she's a woman, a baby may grow. This is her womb (uterus). The womb opens at the bottom, through a small hole called the cervix, into her vagina. At each side

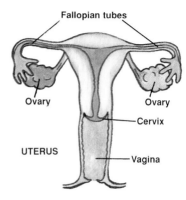

of the top of the womb, two long narrow tubes curve away outwards towards two small blobs.

The tubes are called fallopian tubes, and the blobs are the ovaries, where the eggs are made.

Nothing here is working yet, it's just waiting quietly until the girl grows into a woman.

WHAT'S SPECIAL ABOUT A BOY'S BODY?

Most of the special parts of a boy's body are outside, between his legs. His penis may or may not have a hood of loose skin around the head, (called the foreskin).

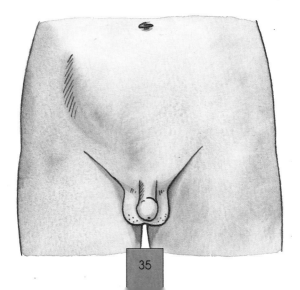

Beneath the penis are two lumps called testicles or balls, inside a bag of skin called the scrotum. When a boy grows up, his testicles will begin to make sperms. The reason why they hang outside his body is because sperms need to be kept cool. The temperature inside a person's body is too hot for sperms to grow properly. When baby boys are born, though, their testicles are tucked inside.

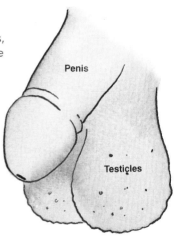

Sometimes, one (or even both) of them may not slip out (descend) into the scrotum by itself when they're supposed to. If this happens it's usually very easy for a doctor to help them to descend.

The testicles are connected to the base of the penis by two very thin tubes which join together and connect up with the tube which carries urine.

Just one tube, called the urethra, travels along the length of the penis. Before a boy grows into a man, this tube only ever carries urine. In a grown-up man, it sometimes carries urine and sometimes sperms, but it's impossible for both to go through at the same time.

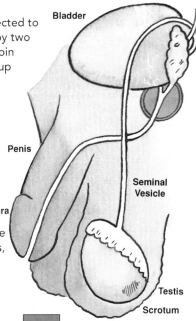

Bladder

Penis

Seminal Vesicle

Urethra

Testis

Scrotum

WHAT IS CIRCUMCISION?

All baby boys are born with a foreskin but it may be removed when the baby boy is very small. This is called circumcision and may be done because of a religious custom or to make the penis easier to keep clean.
If a boy is not circumcised, he must take extra care to clean under his foreskin at bath-time. A boy who is not circumcised can have this small operation after he's grown up if he decides he wants to.

Foreskin

CHANGING SHAPES AND SIZES

Young girls and boys have all the parts they'll need for making babies when they're grown up, but the parts don't start to work until they're ready. There isn't any fixed age when this happens - it could be any time between age 8 and age 18 - but usually girls' bodies begin to grow up, or mature, earlier than boys' bodies.

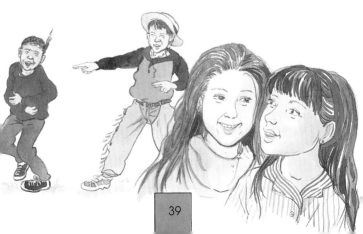

39

ALL CHANGE!

Whenever it happens, though, it can be a surprise. The body that a person has got used to suddenly starts to change. Sometimes this is a welcome change, and sometimes it seems like a nuisance. It can even feel great one day and terrible the next day.

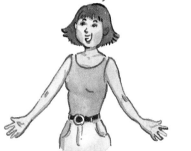 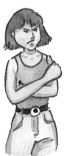

All the changes, and the feelings that go with them, are due to our brand-new sex hormones starting to work. Boys' sex hormones are made in their testicles, and girls' sex hormones are made in their ovaries.

GROWING UP - SLOWLY

When their ovaries or testicles start working, they begin to make the sex hormones which help girls and boys to become grown-up women and men. There's a lot to do, though, and it can take several years.

One of the earliest signs of a boy growing up is when his voice breaks, and one of the earliest things that happens to a girl is that she starts to grow breasts.

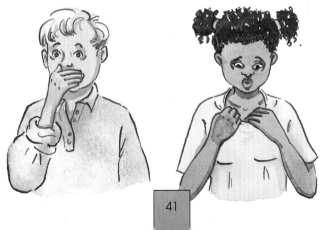

SHAPES AND SIZES

As well as having breasts, the whole shape of a woman's body is different from the shape of a man's body. Growing up affects the whole of a person's body. Girls' bodies become curvy, with wider hip-bones and extra softness over the hips and buttocks (bottom). Their legs and arms grow rounder and smoother, and the rest of their body also becomes less bony-looking.

Boys' bodies become bigger and heavier. Their shoulders grow broader, their arms and legs grow bigger muscles, but their hips and buttocks stay small and firm.

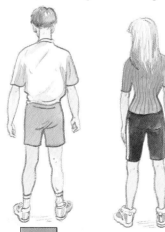

DO SIZE AND SHAPE MATTER?

Changes in shape don't all happen at once, and they don't even happen gradually and steadily. Some boys grow broad-shouldered or tall before their friends do, and then have to wait for the others to catch up; some boys don't start growing bigger until everybody else has finished, but they could eventually grow biggest of all. Some boys grow a bit, then stop, and then grow some more. The way girls grow up is nearly as bumpy as it is for boys.

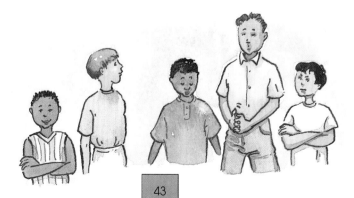

There isn't any shape or size that is 'right' or 'wrong', and there's no 'correct' shape or size for any separate part of a person's body, either. One of the things that makes everybody special is that no two people are the same.

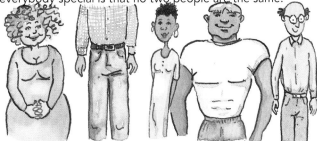

This includes the shapes and sizes of the sexual parts of a boy's body and a girl's body. The size and shape of a woman's breasts is part of her very own special self. The size and shape of a man's penis is a part of his special self. There is no 'correct' shape for these or any other sexual parts - it's just another way people are different.

WHAT ARE HORMONES?

Hormones are powerful chemicals, made by several glands in your body, which can cause a lot of different things to happen all at once.

One kind of hormone, called adrenaline, which comes from two tiny glands near your kidneys, is made whenever you get a fright. It makes your body get ready, all in a flash, to cope with danger. It may help you to run away, or to fight. It makes you breathe faster and makes your heart beat more quickly; it can make you go pale, too, and may make you tremble.

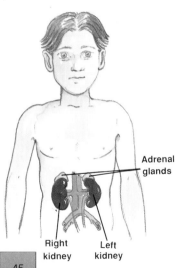

Adrenal glands

Right kidney

Left kidney

When your ovaries (if you're a girl) or testicles (if you're a boy) begin working to make eggs and sperms, they also start making new sex hormones. Sex hormones cause a lot of the body changes that happen when girls and boys grow up.

They can also set off other hormones, including adrenaline, which is one reason why adolescence can be a time when tears and tempers can suddenly come and go.

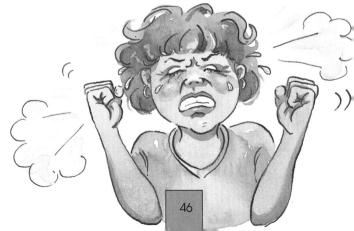

TEARS, TEMPERS, BLUSHES AND ZITS

It takes a little time for newly-started ovaries or testes to get properly organised. To begin with, things don't always go smoothly. Because hormones can affect a person's moods as well as their body, during adolescence, when their sex hormones are still getting their act together, they can sometimes change very quickly from feeling fine to feeling really miserable or angry, without any real reason.

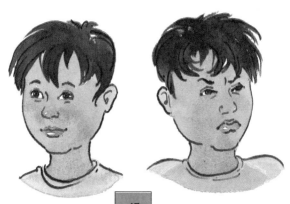

For some people, this may be a time when they feel angry, unhappy, shy, self-conscious or easily embarrassed. These feelings may seem very strong when they come, and can even upset relationships with friends, family or teachers, but they don't last very long.

Zits are another problem caused by disorganised sex hormones. Nearly everybody has them when they're growing up, but they go away, too, when the sex hormones settle down.

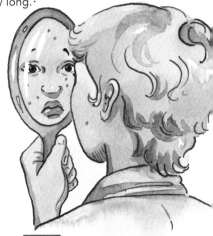

WHY DO GIRLS GROW BREASTS?

Both girls and boys have nipples, but a boy's nipples stay flat even when he grows up. When a girl begins to become a woman, she may notice that her nipples swell up and feel sore. This feeling can come and go several times, before her breasts start to grow properly. The age when this happens isn't any particular time.

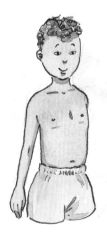
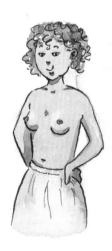

Everybody is different in other ways, and girls can be very different in this way, too. Eventually, a girl's breasts will reach the size they are meant to be for her and then they will stop growing. It doesn't matter what size or shape they are.

What they're there for is to make milk to feed a baby, one day when the girl is a woman.

Although all female mammals have breasts for feeding their babies, hardly any of them have to carry swollen ones around when they haven't got a baby to feed.

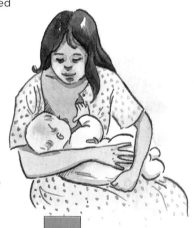

THE RIGHT EQUIPMENT

If a girl finds her breasts suddenly seem to get in the way, it's probably time to give them some support with a bra.

When choosing a bra, there are two different measurements to look at. One measurement is chest size, and this will be the same as the size of all the girl's other clothes. The other measurement is cup size, and this helps to match the bra with the size of the breasts themselves. The smallest cup size is AA, the next size is A and the largest size is DD. A sports bra gives the best support for playing games.

51

FOR BOYS TOO

A boy may also find he needs some support and protection for his penis and testicles when playing sports. For most sports, a jock strap helps to prevent these parts from jigging about and getting in the way. For cricket, boys and men wear a hard protective box to keep their penis and testicles safe in case they're hit by the hard ball.

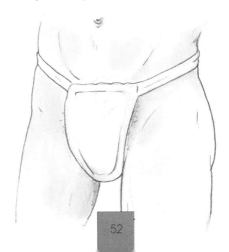

BODY HAIR - THE LOWDOWN

WHY, WHERE, AND WHEN DO WE GROW BODY HAIR?

When our sex hormones start working, they've got a lot of work to do. First, they have to cause all the changes that turn a boy into a man, or a girl into a woman. One of the differences between children and grown-ups is that grown-ups have hair growing on other parts of their body as well as their head.

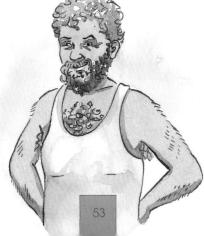

53

HERE...

Adolescent boys and girls begin to grow hair in their armpits, where their arms join their body. This is a place where we sweat a lot, and one of the reasons for having hair here is connected with sweating. Sweat can change its odour (smell) to carry messages through the air - it can tell other people if you are angry, or afraid. When you're grown-up, it can also tell other people if you are feeling sexy.

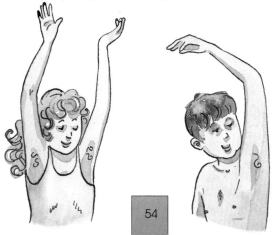

The hair in your armpit probably helps these odours to spread into the air to send their messages. Some people think that the odour of sweat isn't nice so they use deodorants to take the odour away. If your body is clean, though, your sweat has practically no odour at all.

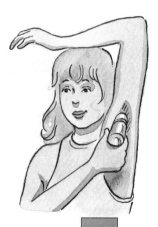

Hair also grows around the sexual parts of men and women. This is called pubic hair. Pubic hair is curly, even if the hair on your head is straight. The patch of pubic hair a woman has is usually a neater shape than the pubic hair that grows around the base of a man's penis. Like everything else about people, the pattern of pubic hair is different for everybody. Some people grow a lot, others grow less, some people have a big patch and others have a small one. This is something you inherit from your parents, and it really doesn't matter at all what pattern of pubic hair your body decides to grow.

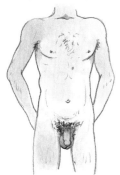
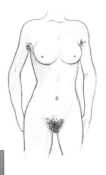

56

...EVERYWHERE!

As well as growing hair in the same places as women, men may also grow more hair on their whole body. It can become especially thick on their chest, arms and legs, and sometimes on their shoulders. And, of course, men grow hair on their face.

The amount of body or facial hair each man grows is as different from other men as everything else about him. Some men grow a lot and some grow hardly any at all. It really doesn't matter how much or how little body or facial hair a man - or a woman - has.

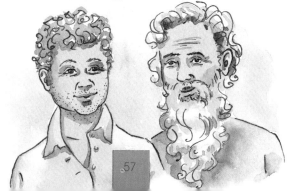

Both men and women can choose whether to let their hair grow as much as it wants to, or whether to cut it or shave it off altogether. Men can choose whether to grow a beard or shave their face; women often choose to shave (or use creams) to remove the hair under their armpits and on their legs. If any hair is shaved or creamed away, when it grows back again it will feel thicker and more prickly because all the fine, silky ends have been chopped off.

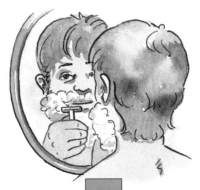

WHY DOES A BOY'S VOICE BREAK?

Boys' and girls' voices sound very much alike. Men's and women's voices, though, are very easy to tell apart. It's not the girl's voice that changes, but the boy's, and it happens very suddenly. When it first starts, a boy's voice can become very hard to control for a short while.

While a boy's voice is breaking, it may sometimes come out like the boy's voice he's used to, and sometimes like a strange new man, and might even change in the middle of a single word. This can be embarrassing, but is only a real nuisance for a boy who has been a singer, because he suddenly has to stop singing altogether until his voice settles down into the new man's voice he will have for the rest of his life.

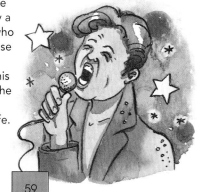

Nobody can tell whether a boy singer is going to become a grown-up tenor, baritone or bass until it happens.

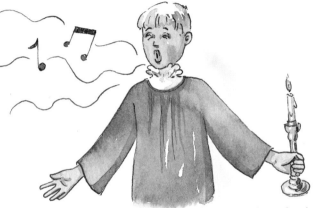

But the real reason a boy's voice changes isn't so that he can sing differently. It's a sign that his body is growing up into a man, and his testicles are beginning to make hormones.

WHAT IS AN ERECTION?

A man's penis is usually soft and floppy, but when it gets ready to put sperms into a woman's vagina it becomes stiff and firm. When a man's penis becomes stiff, this is called 'having an erection', because it also stands erect.

Sometimes, an erection can happen just from looking at a girl or woman and having a sexy thought. This can be embarrassing, but it is quite normal and happens to all boys and men sometimes.

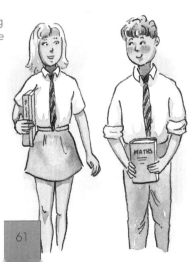

Because sperms and urine can't come out of a penis at the same time, it's practically impossible for a boy to urinate while he has an erection.

WHAT ARE WET DREAMS?

When a boy's testicles start working, making sperms and sex hormones, they also give him sexy feelings and erections. These often begin to happen just at night, in his dreams. If a boy has a sexy dream, he may have an erection, and some sperms and fluid (semen) may even come out of his penis while he's asleep. When he wakes up he might not remember the dream at all, but his pyjamas or sheets might still be wet from the semen which came out while he was dreaming.

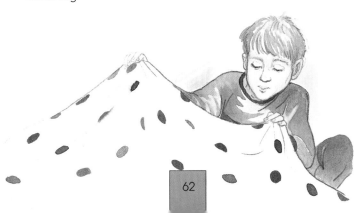

This happens to every boy when he is growing up.
It happened to every grown-up man you know, and it
often goes on happening right through a man's life. It is
another sign that a boy's body is beginning to work like
a man's body.

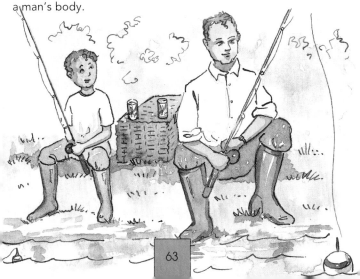

DO GIRLS HAVE WET DREAMS?

Girls can have sexy dreams, just as boys do. They are caused by girls' sex hormones. A girl's body also makes some fluid when she feels sexy but, because a girl's body doesn't make nearly as much fluid as a boy's does, when she wakes up she might not notice that this has happened.

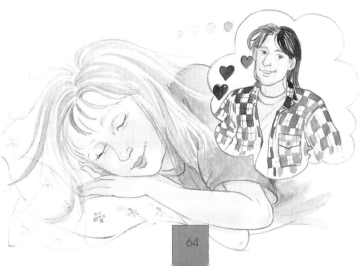

WHO, WHEN, WHERE?

Anybody can have sexy feelings, even when they are alone and doing nothing special. When this happens to a boy, his penis may become stiff (erect) and ticklish. An erect penis likes to be touched, and so it's hard not to stroke it when this happens. This is called masturbating or playing with yourself, and most boys and men do it sometimes.

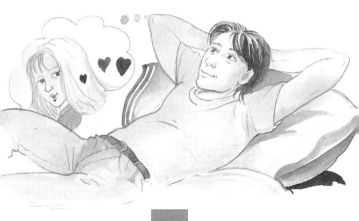

When a girl has sexy feelings, her clitoris (the tiny lump at the front of her vulva) can also grow bigger and become hard (erect). An erect clitoris also likes to be stroked, and so girls and women sometimes masturbate, too. Because a girl's clitoris is similar to a man's penis, it's also very hard for a girl to urinate if her clitoris is erect.

Masturbating is something people do by themselves, so it's not the same as having sex or making love. Like all the other things people do, it's not a problem unless it gets in the way of other things in your life. This is a very private matter.

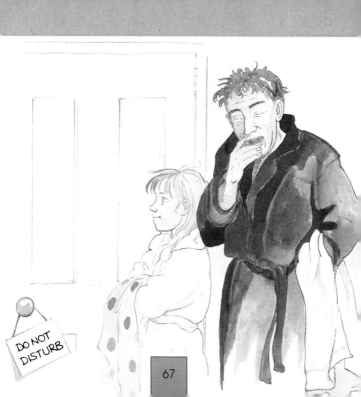

DO NOT DISTURB

WHAT ARE PERIODS?

One of the things that happen when a girl begins to change into a woman is that her womb starts to work. The first sign of this is when, one day, a little bit of blood comes out of her vagina. It's always a surprise, because nobody ever knows when it will happen. It has usually started happening by the time a girl is 15, but it can begin as early as age 10.

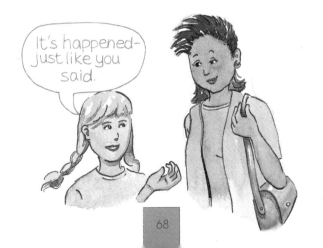

All grown-up women get used to this happening, for three, four or even five days every single month of their life, until they get to the age of about 50. Because it happens so regularly, it is called a period. (The other name, menstruation, comes from the Latin for 'month'.)

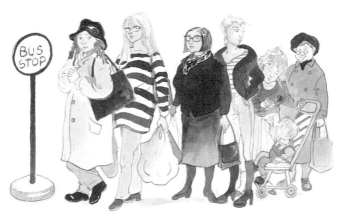

DON'T PANIC!

When it first starts happening, though, it isn't usually regular at all. After the first time, several months could go by before it happens again. This can be a difficult time for a girl, because if she doesn't know when to expect her period to come, it's hard for her to be ready to keep the blood from staining her pants or the sheets on the bed. But every girl can be sure that all the grown-up women that she knows had the same difficult time, years ago when they started growing up. Her mother will understand the problem and help her to cope with it.

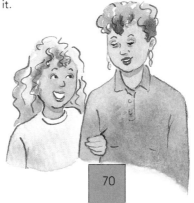

There are two main ways that a woman can keep the blood from her period from staining her pants. One way is to put a soft pad (towel) inside her pants to soak up the blood as it comes out. After a little practice, it's quite easy to tell when the pad needs to be thrown away and replaced with a new, dry one.

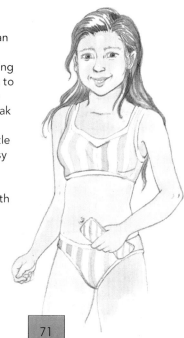

There are lots of different types and shapes of pads to choose from, because every woman in the world needs them, every month of the year, for 40 years of her life. Grown-up women sometimes use a specially shaped pad, a thin cylinder called a tampon, which goes right inside their vagina. This soaks up the blood before it even comes out. It's best for a girl not to try using one of these to begin with, though, because her body still has some more growing and changing to do.

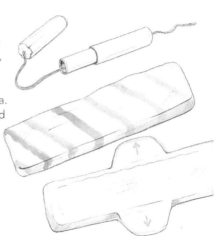

So far, having a period seems to be nothing but a lot of trouble. But that's only on the outside. What it really means is that, inside, a girl's baby-making parts are starting to work.

When she starts to have periods, it means that a girl's body can also make and grow a baby, even though the rest of her isn't ready to do this yet.

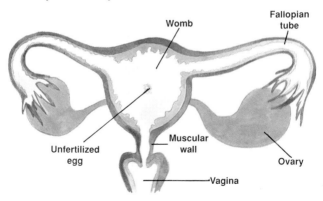

Womb

Fallopian tube

Unfertilized egg

Muscular wall

Ovary

Vagina

WHAT CAUSES PERIODS?

Inside a woman's body, her two ovaries are full of growing eggs. Each month, one egg grows bigger until it is ripe and ready to slip away from the ovary and start its journey down the tube that leads to the womb. While this is happening the womb is getting ready, in case the egg gets fertilised and starts to grow into a baby.

This cannot happen, of course, unless a man has put some sperms into the woman's vagina, because an egg by itself is only half of what makes a baby. The other half has to come from a man's sperm.

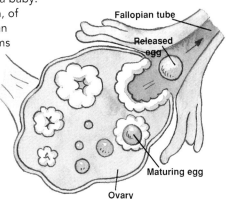

Fallopian tube

Released egg

Maturing egg

Ovary

But the womb doesn't know what's going to happen so it gets ready, every time an egg is ready, just in case the egg happens to be fertilised this time.

Every month, then, a woman's womb grows a thick, soft, cushiony lining. The tiny veins there become fatter, in case they will be needed to bring blood to feed a growing baby.

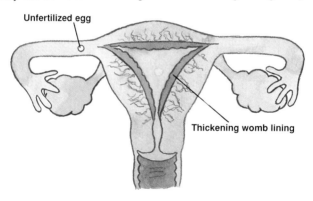

Unfertilized egg

Thickening womb lining

TWENTY EIGHT DAYS TO GO

When the egg doesn't get fertilised by a sperm (which is nearly always), the womb simply throws away that thick, soft lining and starts to grow a new one for the next egg. When the cast-off lining comes out of a woman's vagina, it causes the little bit of bleeding called a period. The shortest time it can take between one egg ripening and the next one to be ready is four weeks, and this is why a woman usually has her periods four weeks apart.

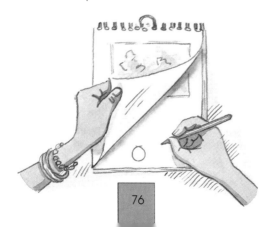

EXERCISE HELPS... HONESTLY!

Sometimes having a period can hurt a bit, because the womb's lining doesn't come off as easily as usual. Some girls can get quite unpleasant period pains during the first day or two, especially when their periods have only recently begun.

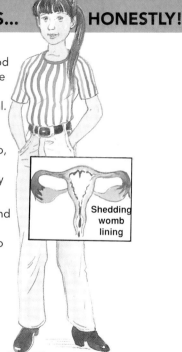

Shedding womb lining

It often helps to go out and take a brisk run, or jog or skip, because this helps to unstick the womb lining, although it might be the last thing anyone would feel like doing when they have a period pain!

HALFWAY THROUGH

Some women even have a tiny twinge at the very moment that an egg slips from one of their ovaries, but most women don't feel anything at all to tell them when this is happening. The actual moment when a ripe egg leaves an ovary is about halfway between two periods, in other words, two weeks after the last period began. This is the time when a woman can most easily start making a baby (become pregnant).

MAY

S	M	T	W	T	F	S
	1	2	3	4	5	6
7	8	9	10	11	12	13
14	15	16	17	18	19	20
21	22	23	24	25	26	27
28	29	30	31			

JUNE

S	M	T	W	T	F	S
				1	2	3
4	5	6	7	8	9	10
11	12	13	14	15	16	17
18	19	20	21	22	23	24
25	26	27	28	29	30	

X – Period
◯ – Egg released

78

BOYS AND GIRLS TOGETHER

WHY DO BOYS AND GIRLS START GOING OUT TOGETHER?

When boys and girls start going out together, they do it because they want to, because it's fun for a boy to be with a girl and it's fun for a girl to be with a boy. They may enjoy just being together, like all friends do, but they may also get a specially good feeling about being with a special friend of the opposite sex. This new feeling might make them want to hold hands. When they know one another better and are sure they really like and trust one another, they may want to kiss and hug and touch one another's bodies, too.

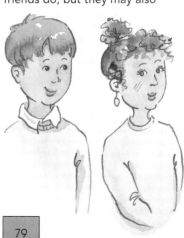

SO MUCH TO LEARN

The time when boys and girls suddenly start wanting to go out together is around the time that their sex hormones are starting to work. As well as changing a person's body, sex hormones also affect our feelings. So when boys and girls start to grow up, they also begin to feel like grown-up men and women who may, one day, decide to live together and make a baby. But there's still a lot to learn about these new feelings, just as there's a lot to learn about living in a new, grown-up body.

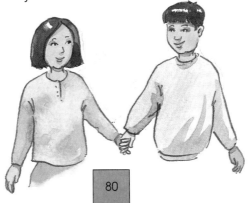

The reason why men and women enjoy playing with one another's bodies is because it is meant to be fun, when we are ready and when we are sure we want to. In one way, it's easy to explain why it's fun - it simply has to be fun because nobody would ever have babies if what you had to do to make a baby was something dreadful, or even if it was just plain boring.

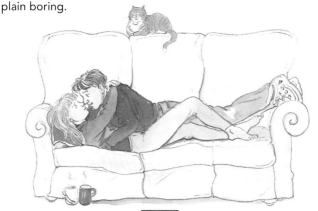

It's important to understand that the pleasure that boys and girls can give to each other is really part of nature's trick to make sure that new babies are started. The attraction between a man and a woman is nature's crafty way of bringing them together so that an egg and a sperm can meet.

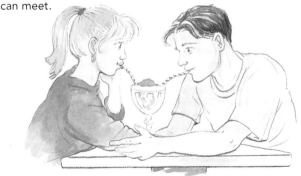

Nature makes it pleasant for us to do everything else we have to do, too, like eating to keep alive.

HOW DO WE LEARN TO CONTROL STRONG FEELINGS?

If you're hungry, it's sometimes very hard to wait even a few more minutes until dinner-time. This is because, as well as getting pleasure from eating, there is also a force, called your appetite, which makes you want to eat. But you know that just stuffing something into your mouth the moment you want to eat can be greedy, or selfish, or silly, or even dangerous. And it's the same with sex.

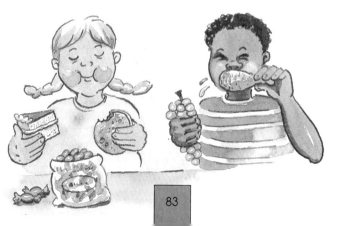

TAKE YOUR TIME

It may be very hard to resist, especially when it's a new feeling which you haven't got used to yet. You've been learning how to feed yourself since you were a baby, after all (and what a mess you made of that, too, when you first started!), and this powerful new drive or appetite is 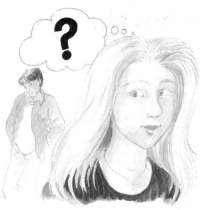 going to take some handling. There's a lot more to learn about sex than about food. It will take quite a long time to learn all you need to know, so it makes sense to take it slowly, and find out the best and safest ways to enjoy all the good things that boys and girls, or men and women, can do together.

Unlike eating, making love is something which two people do together. It is the most special, most personal, and closest thing which two people can do together. If two people don't take care to understand and respect one another's feelings, and truly trust each other, making love can be a bad experience for one or both of them.

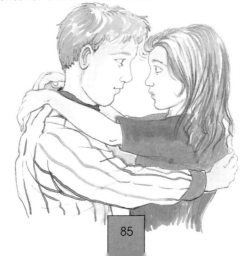

WHAT DOES BEING IN LOVE MEAN?

When a boy and a girl like one another so much that just being together can make them both feel very happy, and being apart can make them feel sad, then they are probably in love. Being in love can be wonderful, but there are times when it can also seem very hard.

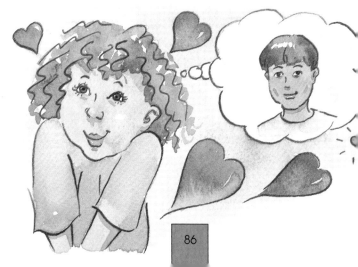

NOT JUST ONE-SIDED

Sometimes, one person can have very strong feelings, all alone, about another person. This is called 'infatuation' or a crush, and it can be very painful for the person who has those feelings. It could even give the other person a chance to hurt them if they decided to. Hurting another person is always wrong, but hurting somebody who cares for you is one of the cruellest things anyone can do.

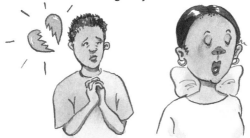

Even when two people love each other, they must take special care not to be hurtful, and not make each other do things they don't want to do.

WHAT DOES 'MAKING LOVE' MEAN?

Making love means giving pleasure to, and enjoying the body of, somebody you love and who loves you. It does not have to mean the same as 'having sex'. It can mean sending romantic letters, kissing, cuddling, or touching one another in any way which pleases both partners. But if something doesn't feel absolutely right - before it happens, or when it's happening, or even afterwards - then there is a risk that it could spoil a good friendship.

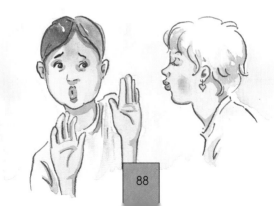

TALK ABOUT IT

Two people who really love one another, and who are grown-up, or mature enough to handle it will also want to talk to each other and understand one another's feelings.

Talking is another way of sharing. Starting to talk may be difficult but, once you begin, it becomes much easier. The only way to find out what somebody else thinks or feels is to ask them. Talking about feelings can also help you to work out what you feel.

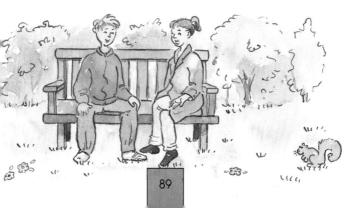

WHAT DOES 'HAVING SEX' MEAN?

Having sex means two people putting their sex parts (penis; vagina) as close as they can. It is also called 'going all the way' and 'penetration'. Even if a man's penis doesn't go inside a woman's vagina, if they come close enough together they could still start a baby.

Men and women can enjoy making love without doing this.

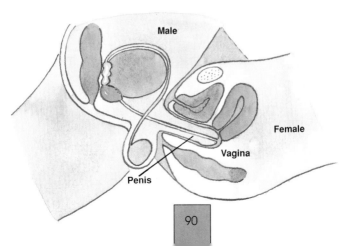

WHAT DOES BEING GAY MEAN?

Nobody can choose their eye colour, or how tall they grow. And nobody can choose who they will be sexually attracted to, either. Some people are naturally attracted to people of the opposite sex; we say they are heterosexual or 'straight'.

Some people are naturally attracted to people who are the same sex as they are; we say they are homosexual or gay. Gay women are sometimes also called lesbians.

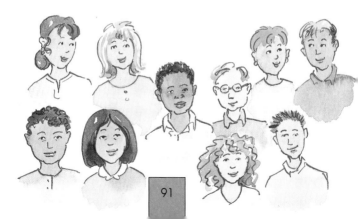

Everyone has friends who are the same sex as themselves, but this does not mean that everybody is gay. The number of people who do grow up to be truly gay might be around one in ten. Sometime or another, both girls and boys may have quite strong sexual feelings towards people of the same sex as themselves, especially during the time when their new sex hormones are settling down.

Young people sometimes feel this way, for a short time, about somebody older. This is called having a crush, and doesn't mean that they will grow up to be gay. If it did, then the number of gay grown-ups would be a lot more than one in ten!

There are even more people, called bisexual, who can be sexually attracted to both men and women. A person's choice of sexual partner is a very personal and private thing. It doesn't affect the way he or she makes friends with other people.

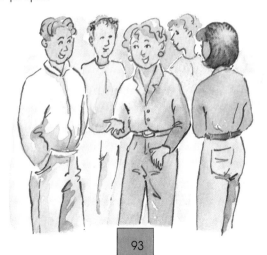

WHEN TO SAY 'NO'

Making love does not mean one person doing things to another person which the other person does not want them to do. Having sex is not something you do to prove that you trust somebody, but something you don't do unless you trust somebody. If one person tells another person to have sex with them, or forces them to do it, this is wrong. It's so wrong that it is against the law to make somebody have sex if they don't want to do it.

This is a serious crime called rape.

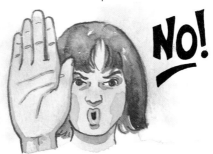

It is against the law for a grown-up person to have sex with a person younger than 16 years old. This is called abuse. It is also against the law for a person to do anything connected with sex parts (especially penis; vagina), or even to show them off to another person who doesn't want them to. This is called indecency.

Anyone who feels someone has done one of these things to them should tell somebody else about it.

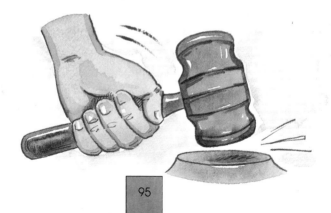

WHAT DOES 'SAFE SEX' MEAN?

'Safe sex' means taking care not to pass on, or catch a disease from someone else through having sex with them. Just as it's possible to catch a cold from someone else's sneeze, it is also possible to catch one of a small number of diseases by having sex with someone who has the disease.

These diseases are called sexually transmitted diseases (STDs). There are several different STDs, and each one can make a person ill in a different way. But there is one way to guard against giving or catching all of them.

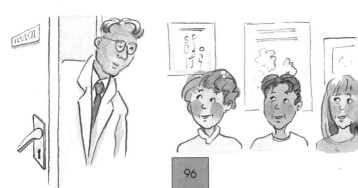

96

CONDOMS

If a man always fits a thin rubber skin, called a condom or sheath, over his penis before having sex, this protects both partners from infection because it will be impossible for any disease to get in or out.

'Safe sex' means always using a new, clean condom. It is very easy for anybody to buy condoms from all chemists shops and some other shops. Some Health Centres and Family Planning Clinics even give them away, free. Clinics can also give other help and advice, and have leaflets to take away and books to read.

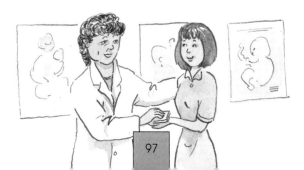

WHAT IS A CONTRACEPTIVE?

When people make love or have sex, they don't always want to make a baby. Choosing to make a baby is a big decision, because it means that a new person will be born, who will need to be loved and cared for until he or she grows up. But making love is something that two people who love one another can enjoy doing together, even if they don't want to make a baby.

A contraceptive is the name we give to any of the different things people can use to prevent a baby being made when they have sex.

There are a lot of different contraceptives to choose from. They include 'the pill'; the diaphragm or Dutch cap; the coil or IUD; and the 'safe period'. But none of these methods is the same as safe sex. The only contraceptive which is also 'safe' in every other way is the condom. (See also page 175.)

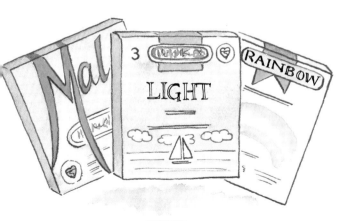

WHAT ARE HIV AND AIDS?

HIV is a virus disease which can be caught or given through having sex, and also by doing other things which might allow two people's blood to meet. Unlike most other sexually transmitted diseases (STDs), it can take many years for a person to find out if he or she has caught the HIV virus. This means that anybody who has ever had unsafe sex (or done something else which has let their blood meet another person's blood) could have caught the virus, and could give it to other people, without knowing it.

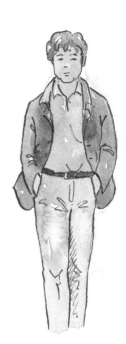

100

Although the HIV virus doesn't make a person ill for a long, long time, it slowly works inside their body until the signs of illness called AIDS begin to show. In other words, HIV causes AIDS. HIV can be in a person's body for up to ten years (perhaps even longer) before AIDS starts to show, but once AIDS starts (and as far as we know, it always does, sooner or later) it leads to death. So far, nobody has discovered a cure for HIV or AIDS.

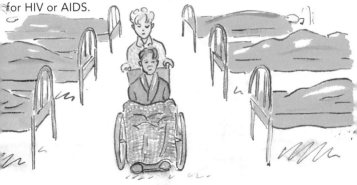

Because this is such a dangerous disease, and so hard to detect, it really means that using a condom is the only sensible and responsible way to have sex, especially with a new partner. Partners who care about each other will naturally want to take care not to harm one another. If one of them doesn't want to bother with a condom, it could be a sign that this person isn't worth bothering with.

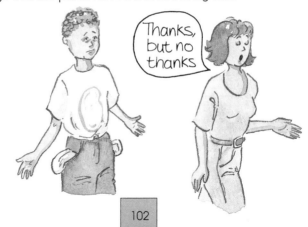

People who have been unlucky enough to catch HIV cannot give the disease to other people in any way except through unsafe sex or their fresh blood. It is perfectly safe to touch somebody with HIV or AIDS, or their belongings, and to share the same bathroom, the same kitchen, and the same cups and knives and forks, as long as the person isn't bleeding.

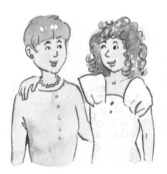

MAKING A BABY

HOW DO A MAN'S SPERMS GET INSIDE A WOMAN'S BODY?

When a man and a woman have decided they want to make a baby, they begin by cuddling up very close and kissing and stroking one another. This is called foreplay. It is probably something they have done together lots of times already as part of making love, before they decided to try to make a baby, so they already know what they like to do best.

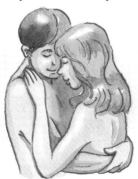

Soon, the man's penis will change from being small and soft. It will grow bigger, and become stiff and hard. When this happens, it doesn't hang down any more but points upwards. This is called an erection, and has happened to the man lots of times before.

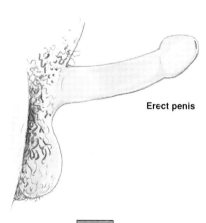

Erect penis

Kissing and cuddling makes a woman's vagina wet and slippery, too. So when both of them are ready, it is easy for the man to slip his penis gently inside the woman's vagina. This is very nice for both of them, and makes them want to rub their penis and vagina together. The rubbing movement makes the semen, which contains the man's sperms, spurt out of his penis into the woman's vagina, all at once. This is called having an orgasm, or 'coming', or reaching a climax.

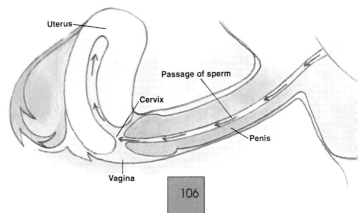

Uterus

Passage of sperm

Cervix

Penis

Vagina

For a woman, having an orgasm means her vagina pulsates (throbs), which helps to pull the man's semen into her womb. When a couple want to make a baby, of course, they want a sperm and an egg to meet so they don't use any method of birth control (contraception).

After a man and a woman have made love they feel very relaxed and happy together and they may feel sleepy, too.

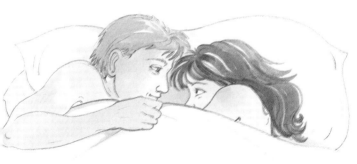

HOW DO THE EGG AND THE SPERM MEET?

A man's semen contains millions and millions of tiny sperms, which look a bit like tadpoles. Each one has a tiny head (filled with half of the man's own chromosomes) and a long wriggly tail (for swimming). All the sperms start to swim up the woman's vagina, in a great race. They race right through the cervix, through the womb, and up the fallopian tubes. If there is an egg in one of the tubes, just ready to be fertilised, the first sperm to get there wriggles right inside the egg and the race is over. The outside of the egg changes, very quickly, so that any other sperms which manage to get that far simply can't get in.

Inside the egg, the father's half-set of chromosomes (brought by the sperm which won the race) add themselves to the mother's half-set of chromosomes (which were already there), and the whole new code for a brand-new person is made.

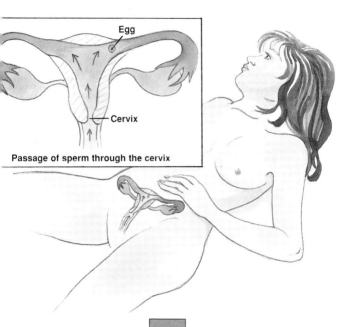

Egg

Cervix

Passage of sperm through the cervix

HOW DOES THE EGG START TO GROW?

When an egg has been fertilised, it starts to grow from just one cell into the 200 million cells which make up the body of a new baby. This begins slowly, and then goes more and more quickly. First of all, the egg splits in two. This is how one cell becomes two cells. Each of these two cells then splits into two (making 4), and the four new cells split again (making 8). The cells split over and over again until there are enough of them to turn into a hollow ball made of hundreds of cells.

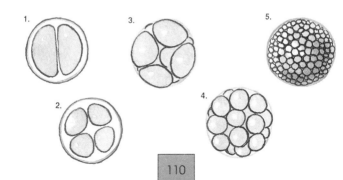

1.

2.

3.

4.

5.

During the week or so while this is happening, the growing ball of cells floats gently down the fallopian tube to the mother's womb.

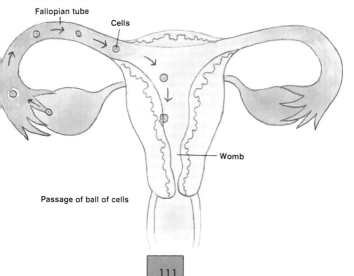

Fallopian tube

Cells

Womb

Passage of ball of cells

HOW DOES A WOMAN KNOW...

...IF SHE HAS STARTED GROWING A BABY?

When a baby starts to grow inside her womb, the first sign a mother has is that her periods stop. They must stop, of course, because they are only caused by her womb lining coming out when a baby hasn't started growing there. For as long as the baby needs to live inside her womb, the lining stays firmly fixed and a woman has no periods.

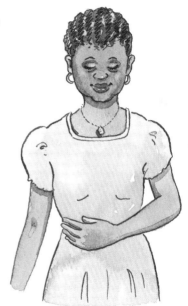

But there can be other reasons why a woman's periods may stop, so the next thing she will do is to have a pregnancy test. This can be done very easily - even using a kit which she can buy at the chemist's shop - but she will probably go to see her doctor when she thinks she might be pregnant. The doctor can then give her some advice about what happens next, and how to care for herself and the new baby growing inside her.

Growing a baby, from the moment the sperm fertilises the egg to the day the baby is born, takes between 38 and 40 weeks.

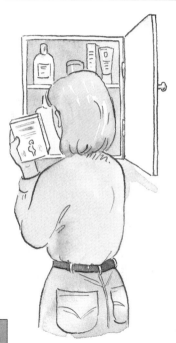

113

The tiny ball of cells floats into the womb and sinks deep into the soft lining. Little tentacles grow out all around it and burrow into the lining, mingling with the swollen veins there.

This is where the baby's food, and other things it needs to live and grow, will come from until it is born. The food and other things leak out of mother's blood into baby's blood. Mother's blood also carries away the wastes from the baby's body.

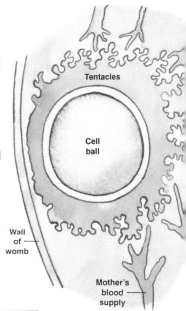

Tentacles

Cell ball

Wall of womb

Mother's blood supply

114

The baby soon grows too big to stay buried in the wall of the womb. It gradually bulges out more and more into the hollow centre of the womb until only the tentacles are left touching the wall. This part is now called the baby's placenta, and it will stay 'plugged in', collecting supplies from mother's blood, until the baby is born. The baby is connected to its placenta by a cord of veins, called the umbilical cord.

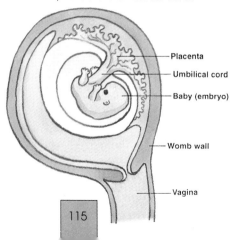

Placenta

Umbilical cord

Baby (embryo)

Womb wall

Vagina

THE BABY'S FIRST THREE MONTHS

The most important time in the baby's whole life is the first three months inside its mother's womb. In the first three months it goes all the way from being a tiny fertilised egg, too small to see without a microscope, to being a whole new person, complete with fingers and toes. At the end of three months, it is about 5 inches (13 cm) long.

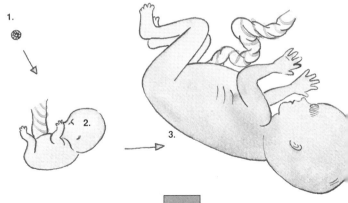

1.

2.

3.

During the first three months of her pregnancy, the baby's mother takes special care not to smoke and not to eat or drink anything which may harm the new baby growing in her womb.

The mother's tummy doesn't look any different yet, because the new baby inside is still very, very small.

THE BABY'S MIDDLE THREE MONTHS

During the second three months of its life the baby just grows and grows. It can't be hurt by all the running and jumping its mother may be doing, because it's floating gently in a bath of lovely warm water (amniotic fluid) inside the womb.

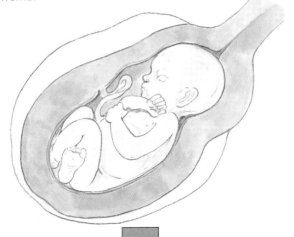

Very soon it starts to do some exercises itself, to help its new muscles to grow strong. It may even start to suck its thumb, to practise for sucking milk after it's born. At the end of this time, it is about 13 inches (33cm) long.

Although most expectant mums can go on living and working and playing as usual, they need to have a rest each day, because the hard work that's going on inside makes them get tired. When the baby does its exercises the mother can feel it moving and kicking inside her, and this is very thrilling.

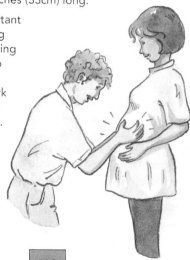

THE BABY'S LAST THREE MONTHS

Now, the baby grows even faster, and the mother's tummy grows bigger every day. The baby is getting ready to be born, to come out of the warm, safe womb into the very different world it will find outside.

Some time during the last three months, the baby usually manages to arrange itself so that its head is at the bottom, ready to come out first.

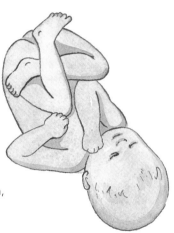

There are some things it can't practise doing yet, like eating and breathing. Inside its mother's womb, the baby doesn't need to breathe or eat with its mouth. As soon as it's born, though, it will have to use its brand-new lungs for the very first time. It will also have to use its mouth to eat for the first time. So, at the same time as it's growing, the baby's lungs and insides are getting ready for the work they'll do for the rest of its long life.

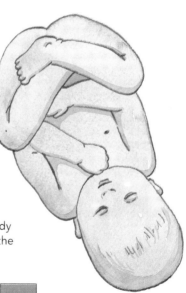

HOW DOES SHE KNOW WHEN IT'S READY

The lessons that she has been having will teach the mother to recognise the signs that her baby is about to be born. She will start to feel her womb grow tight (contract), from time to time, as it begins its exercises for pushing the baby out.

These contractions (labour pains) will begin to come more and more often, as the time for birth gets nearer, and sometimes they can be strong enough to burst the bag of water around the baby. When this happens, she may say that her 'waters have broken'.

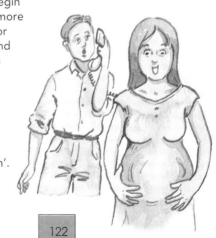

HOW IS A BABY BORN?

The birth of a new baby is very thrilling. There's a lot going on inside the mother's body and inside the baby's body, too, to make the birth happen, and to make sure it's as smooth and simple as it looks.

Inside the mother, the hole the baby will come out of must grow wide enough to allow a baby's head to pass through.

As the time of birth approaches, the opening (cervix) at the bottom of her womb gets bigger and bigger (dilates), and even the bony joint (pubis) in front of her vulva becomes loose. Her vagina is already stretchy enough.

The mother's womb will do most of the work of squeezing the baby out, and to begin with she will try to stay calm and relaxed while this is going on. When the time comes, the mother will help by using her tummy muscles to push, at the same time as the womb squeezes. The midwife will be with her to tell her when it's the right time to do this, and will also be ready to catch (deliver) the baby when it starts to come through the mother's vagina.

The baby's head usually comes out first. This is the biggest and most solid part of the baby, so once the head is delivered the rest of the baby's body slithers out quite easily.

Having a baby always looks very messy. There's a lot of fluid, together with some thin, slippery bits of the bag which contained the fluid, and this comes out at the same time as the baby. Some blood also comes out, but all this is quite normal and is soon cleaned up.

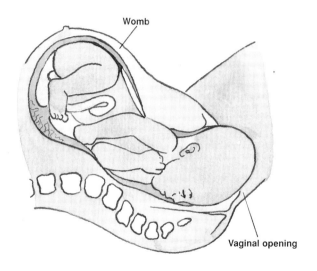

Womb

Vaginal opening

After her baby is born, the mother will be happy but very, very tired. It has been hard work, and might have taken a long time. After she has seen and held her new baby in her arms for the first time, she will probably want to go to sleep.

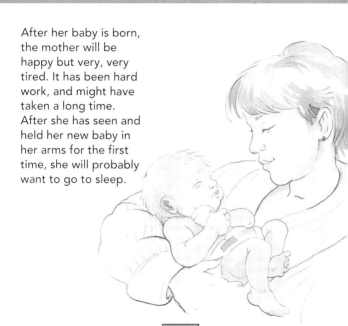

WHAT IS AN AFTERBIRTH?

Afterbirth is another name for the placenta, which was the baby's connection with its mother's womb and brought its food and oxygen while it was growing inside.

It gets its name because it comes out of the womb and slips out of the mother's vagina soon after the baby is born. The baby was attached to its afterbirth (placenta) by the umbilical cord. But after the baby is born this cord isn't needed any longer, so the midwife will tie it tightly and cut it off, close to the baby's tummy.

You still have the little bit of umbilical cord you were left with, in the middle of your tummy. It's called your belly-button.

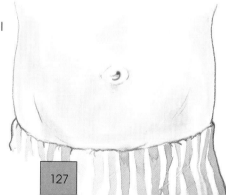

WHY DOES A NEW BABY ALWAYS CRY?

The first thing a new baby has to do is take its very first breath of air. The midwife doesn't wait around for the baby to make up its own mind to start breathing, though. After wiping its nose and mouth clean, she tips it upside-down and gives it a slap on its bottom. So the baby's first breath is often caused by its first big surprise.

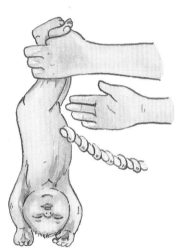

Even if it doesn't need to be helped to start breathing, just being born is a big surprise for a baby who has never been out before, never been cold, never felt air on its skin, and never even seen light. No wonder a new baby always cries!

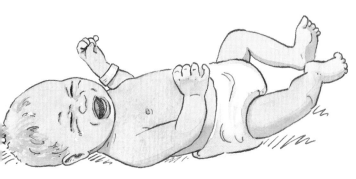

WHAT HAPPENS TO THE NEW BABY?

The baby will be tired, too, after all that squeezing and then the big adventure of seeing and feeling the world for the first time.

When the midwife has made its belly-button, and cleaned it, and when it has been cuddled by its mother and begun to learn her special smell, it will be wrapped up warmly so it can go to sleep.

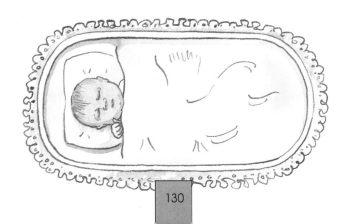

WHAT IS A CAESAREAN BIRTH?

If there is some reason why a mother can't push her baby out of her vagina in the usual way, the doctor may decide to make a hole in the front of her tummy and into her womb to get the baby out that way instead. This is a bit like an ordinary operation to take an appendix out.

The reason it's called a Caesarean birth is because Julius Caesar, the famous Roman Emperor, is supposed to have been the first person to be born this way - over a thousand years ago.

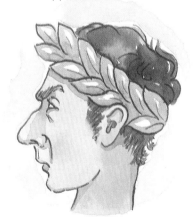

WHAT IS A BREECH BIRTH?

Sometimes, instead of being born head-first, a baby's feet come out first. This is called a breech birth. When this happens, the midwife or doctor may need to give some extra help to the mother and the baby to make sure everything goes smoothly.

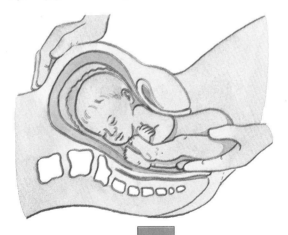

WHAT IS A 'BLUE' BABY?

While the baby was inside its mother's womb, its heart's job was to push all of its blood through the placenta, where all the supplies (including oxygen) came from. When it's born and begins using its own lungs, its heart has to start doing a new job all at once.

Occasionally, a new baby's heart doesn't quite manage this trick. A baby whose heart isn't working perfectly is called a blue baby or hole-in-the-heart baby.

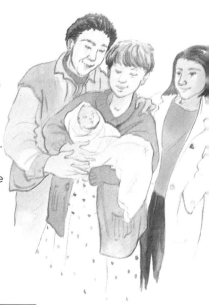

WHAT IS A PREMATURE BABY?

Sometimes, a new baby can be born before it has spent the whole of nine months in its mother's womb. When this happens, it may be called a premature baby. But some of the things that every baby's body needs so that it can live in the cold world outside its mother's warm womb only get finished in the last weeks before it's born. So a premature baby could be born before it was quite ready to be outside.

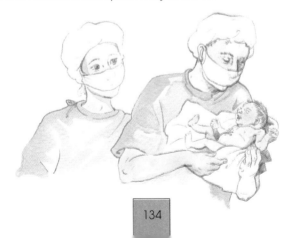

WHAT IS AN INCUBATOR?

An incubator is a special place where a premature baby can get used to being outside its mother's womb before it comes out properly into the cold world. It is a lovely safe, warm, comfortable place, where the baby can be carefully watched over while it finishes growing, until it's safe for it to go home to its family.

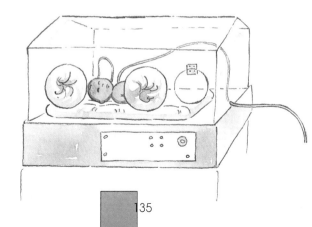

BABY'S WORLD

WHAT DOES A NEW BABY NEED?

A new baby needs warmth, cuddles, milk, sleep and protection from germs. The body of a very new baby can't tell if it's too hot or too cold, so it's important to watch out for these things until the baby is old enough to cry when it's uncomfortable.

To begin with, the baby will spend most of its time asleep, which can be boring for its older brothers and sisters. Very soon, though, it will begin to be more interesting.

WHAT DO NEW BABIES EAT?

New babies get all the food they need from the milk that fills up their mother's breasts. It's nice and warm, and always ready for the baby, whatever its age.

Sometimes, a mother might not want to feed her baby on breast milk, perhaps because she goes out to work and leaves the baby to be cared for by somebody else. Then, she will buy special baby-milk, which will have to be mixed carefully, warmed carefully, and fed to the baby in a carefully-cleaned bottle with a soft nipple-shaped top which it can suck.

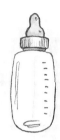

WHY DOES A BABY PUT EVERYTHING INTO ITS MOUTH?

The first real work a baby has to do is suck milk, so it is born with a ready-made habit (instinct) to put things in its mouth. Its lips and tongue are also very sensitive - as yours still are - and help it to 'feel' things in the world before it learns to use its other senses.

Because you can be sure that a baby will try to taste just about everything it can reach, it's important to make sure that everything it can reach is safe to taste and too big to swallow.

TEETHING

Babies are usually born without any teeth. This makes it easier for them to suckle and helps to prevent mother's nipples from getting sore.

Some time in the second six months of its life, the new baby's teeth begin to push through its gums, usually starting with the bottom front teeth. When this is about to happen, the baby may become irritable because its gums are sore.

It takes about two years to grow all twenty teeth. These are called 'milk' teeth, and they only stay for a few years. When the second set of teeth begin to grow, at age 6 or 7, they will push the milk teeth out, one by one.

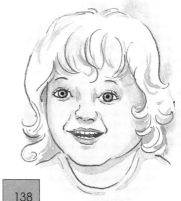

WHEN DO BABIES SLEEP?

For the first three months, the baby will only be awake when it's hungry, about 6 or 8 times in every 24 hours. This goes on through the night, too, so its mother may get very tired during this time.

Gradually, the baby's daytime naps will get shorter and its night-time sleep will become longer, until at last it (and its mother) begins to sleep properly all night.

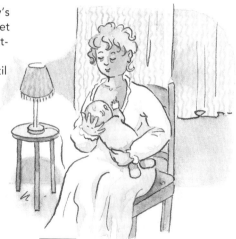

WHY DO BABIES CRY?

Crying is a baby's way of saying 'help!'. This may mean that it's hungry, or that its nappy needs changing. Babies sometimes have wind in their tummy, and this hurts so they cry until somebody picks them up and 'burps' them. They also need a lot of cuddles, and so a baby sometimes cries just because it feels lonely.

If a baby gets too tired, it sometimes can't fall asleep easily. When this happens, rocking the baby in its cradle or pram can help it to relax.

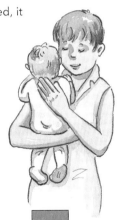

CHANGING NAPPIES

A baby's nappy needs changing just about every time it has a meal, and sometimes in meals. The baby's new, soft skin must be kept clean and dry, so the nappy-changer may use baby powder to dry the skin properly and cream to protect it.

It's safest to lay the baby down on a special mat on the floor to change its nappy, because then it will be in no danger of falling. And it's also important for the nappy-changer's hands to be carefully washed afterwards.

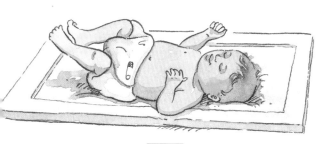

HOW DO BABIES LEARN?

Babies start learning from the first day they're born. But they have such a lot to learn, just to make sense of the world at all, that it might not look as if they're doing much. From the very first moment, though, a baby is working very, very hard.

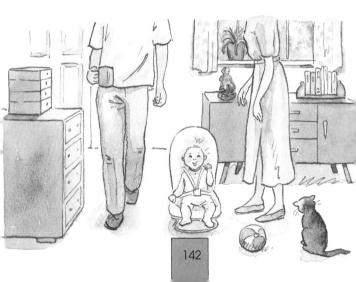

LEARNING TO SEE

To begin with, every baby has blue eyes, and it can only clearly see things which are very close, no more than 20 cm (8 inches) away . During the first few weeks, its eyes gradually begin to see things further away.

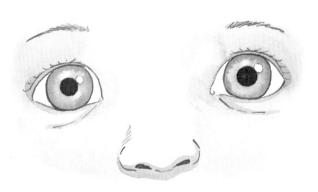

SPECIAL SURROUNDINGS

To a new baby, the most important sight in the world is its mother's smiling face. Other people's smiles are very important, too. The baby won't be able to smile back until it's about six weeks old, but it loves to see everybody else smiling!

When the baby begins gazing at the world all around its cot, it will also enjoy having bright, interesting things to look at. Different colours, different shapes, and things that move will give the baby plenty to study and think about.

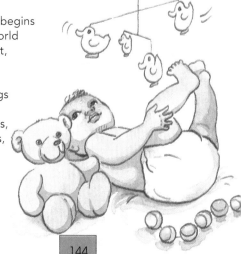

LEARNING TO HEAR AND TALK

Before it was born, the loudest sounds a baby heard inside its mother's womb were the noises made by her body - especially her regular, rhythmic heartbeat. It's not surprising, then, that new babies love to hear music with a good beat.

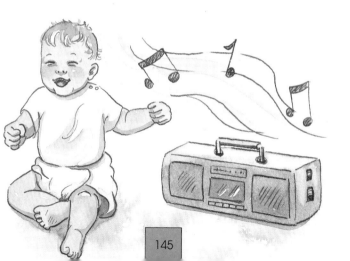

HAPPY TALK

People's voices are important, too. Eventually, the baby will learn to talk just by listening to what people say. So, even before you think a baby can possibly understand you, make sure you talk to it as much as you can. The new baby needs as much help as you can give it.

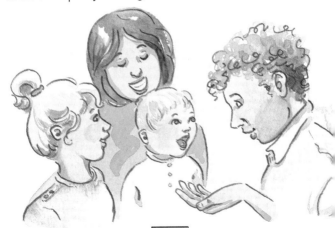

146

LEARNING SKILLS

Between the ages of 3 and 6 months, a baby will reach out to grab at anything that catches its eye. It begins by putting everything into its mouth, and then goes on to practise turning things in its fingers. But it won't be able to pick up anything really small until it's nearly a year old.

Babies quickly learn to get hold of things. But they don't learn to let go for a little while longer, so be patient if a baby offers to give you something and then doesn't seem to want to let it go! In the meantime, the baby will also begin to learn how to fit things together.

It's safest to keep dangerous things out of sight, because a baby can be very clever when it can see something it really wants.

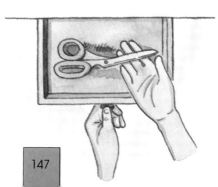

LEARNING TO WALK

Babies learn to crawl about by the time they are around nine months old. Some babies are quite happy to get around like this for a few months, but others are really keen to stand up and walk properly.

Both crawlers and stand-up types will probably learn to walk by themselves soon after their first birthday.

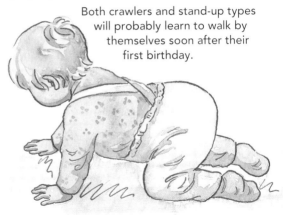

NEW BABY, NEW FAMILY

When a new baby comes into a family, everything changes. Some changes are only for a short time, and some are forever.

Short-term changes are mainly caused by the care and attention a new baby needs. This means that its mother has to think of the baby before she thinks about anything else. If the baby has brothers and sisters, she did this when each of them was a new baby, too .

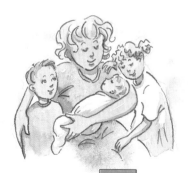

LEND A HAND

Even though they have already had their turn, other members of the family sometimes feel left out or neglected when a new baby arrives. It helps to know that this time doesn't last very long, and also that a baby who gets all the attention he or she needs at the start will be a much nicer person to live with later on. Everybody can help, in some way, to look after the new baby. This will also mean that mother gets less tired and then she will be nicer to live with, too.

The real and forever change, of course, is that there's a new person in the family. Everybody moves up one place, which means that everybody has to get used to a new job. Mother has more people to look after; father has more people to look after; every brother or sister also has more younger people to look after. And the whole family gets a new, special person to turn it into a new and even more special family.

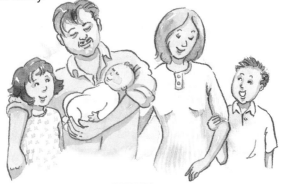

SEX AND CIVILISATION

HOW ARE PEOPLE THE SAME AS OTHER MAMMALS?

All mammal babies start growing inside their mother's body, so all mammal eggs have to be fertilised while they're inside the mother's body. This means that all male mammals have a penis and all female mammals have a vagina.

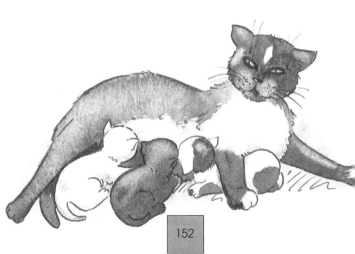

All female mammals, except a very few unusual ones, suckle their babies on milk after they are born. All mammals have some form of courtship before they mate. Some mammals form long relationships with their mates, and some don't.

Some male mammals help the mothers to look after their babies, and some don't. Some mammals live together in families, and some don't. Some mammal babies are born just as helpless as human babies, but some can walk and run almost as soon as they're born.

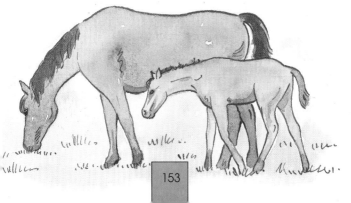

The main sexual difference between people and other mammals is that people do not have a special breeding season. Most other mammals, except a few of the ones that live with us, breed only at special times of the year. At other times, they aren't interested in sex at all.

Many mammal mothers - and not only the meat-eaters - eat some or all of their babies' placentas after they are born.

People also live for a long time after they have stopped being able to have babies. This is probably because we can talk, so the wisdom of older people is very valuable to the rest of the family.

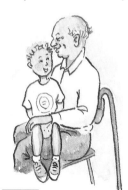

Another difference between people and other mammals is that people think very hard about what they do, and always try to make sense of things that happen. We don't know for sure, of course, but other mammals probably don't worry about sex as much as we do.

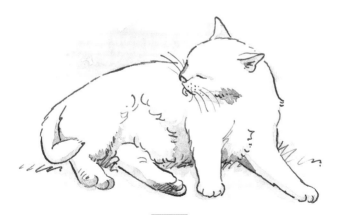

HOW HAS CIVILISATION CHANGED PEOPLE?

We think that the first people were nomads, who spent their lives wandering around in search of food. People like this are called hunter-gatherers. It is a difficult way to live, and is especially hard for a mother with a baby to feed and carry.

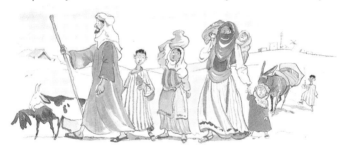

It is possible that hunter-gatherer women did not have 12 chances a year to start a new baby. They probably would not have had a period every month, and perhaps not for a year or even longer. For as long as a mother had one baby to carry, she probably didn't start another one.

Even today, some mothers' periods don't start again until they stop breast-feeding the last baby. This may have been how a woman's body was meant to work, long, long ago.

Even today, some women's periods stop if they are very thin, or if they are very unhappy.

This might also have been useful, long ago, because it could have helped people to survive if they didn't have more babies than they could feed, or if their life was especially hard for other reasons.

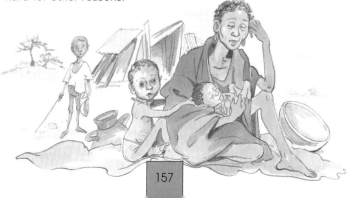

When people learned to plant crops, and to keep special animals for milk and meat, this meant they could settle down and live in one place. Now mothers wouldn't have to walk miles every day carrying their babies, and there would always be plenty to eat. Both of these things could have allowed women to have more babies.

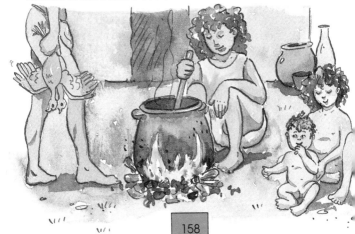

SEXUAL CUSTOMS

DOES EVERYBODY IN THE WORLD HAVE THE SAME SEXUAL CUSTOMS?

People in different parts of the world have a lifestyle which suits the place and way they live. They eat different food, speak different languages, and may also have different sexual customs. Sexual customs can also become part of some people's religion. If they go to live somewhere new, their customs go with them, so even people living in the same town may have different customs.

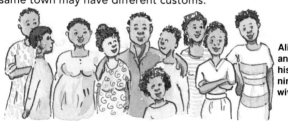

Ali-Begin and his nine wives

Something which is quite ordinary for some people may seem strange to others. This doesn't mean that it is wrong, only that it is different.

The important things in people's lives often have their own special ceremony. When people get married, for instance, the marriage ceremony helps them to tell everybody about their change of lifestyle.

When people grow up, they also start a new lifestyle. Many religions and societies have a special ceremony for this important time. It is a way of telling everyone that this boy or this girl is now a man or a woman, and it helps to make sure that other people stop treating them as if they were still children.

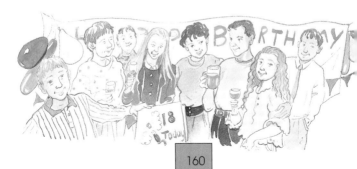

Sometimes, the ceremony includes a special challenge, or trial, which gives the adolescent boy or girl an opportunity to show everyone else that they are truly mature enough to be treated as a grown-up.

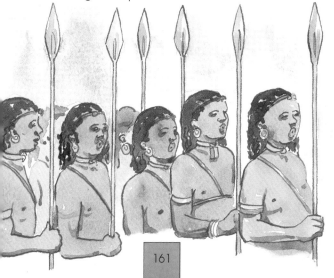

CAN BROTHERS AND SISTERS MARRY ONE ANOTHER?

If a brother and a sister, or a parent and his or her own child, have sex together this is called incest. A long, long time ago, people found out that, if men and women who are closely related have babies together, these babies are much more likely to die or be deformed in some way.

Because of this and other reasons, incest is now absolutely forbidden nearly everywhere in the world.

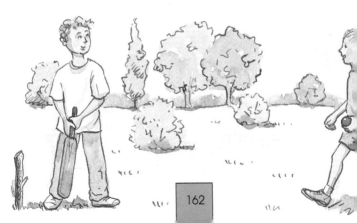

CAN PEOPLE WITH SPECIAL PROBLEMS MAKE LOVE?

Anybody can love someone and be loved by someone. Having a special problem doesn't change a person's sex, or their feelings. Everyone's needs and wishes are different, whether or or not they have a special problem that other people can see, and every single person has to work out their own special way to live their own special life.

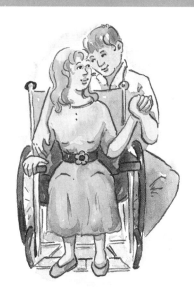

The only way anybody ever finds out if they can have babies is by trying to make a baby when they want to.

WHAT IS A TEST-TUBE BABY?

Occasionally, when two people want to make a baby they may need a little help to get things started. Doctors can sometimes help by taking an egg out of the mother's body and making sure that it is fertilised properly. When the egg has been fertilised, it is put back into the mother's womb to grow there normally.

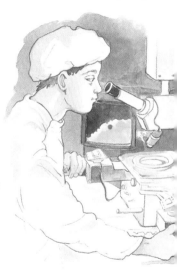

The name 'test-tube baby' doesn't mean that the baby grew in a test-tube, only that it began there, for just a moment. This is just one of the ways doctors can help people to make babies.

FOSTERING AND ADOPTION

WHAT IS THE DIFFERENCE BETWEEN FOSTERING AND ADOPTION?

When two people adopt a baby or child, he or she becomes a permanent part of their family, exactly as a baby of their own would have been from the start. When adopted children grow up, they can choose whether or not to find out about their 'natural' parents.

If there is a reason why a young person's mother or father cannot take care of them, just for a while, then they may be fostered. This means living as part of a new family for as long as the arrangement lasts.

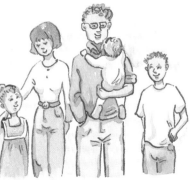

RESPONSIBLE PARENTS

HOW MANY BABIES CAN A WOMAN HAVE?

It takes about nine calendar months (40 weeks) to make a baby. So it's quite possible for a mother to have a baby each year of her life between the time when her ovaries start working and the time when they stop.

This means a mother might have as many as 35 children by the time she was 50 years old. In fact, the world record is held by a Russian mother who lived just over 200 years ago. She had 16 pairs of twins, 7 sets of triplets, and 4 sets of quads, making 69 children altogether!

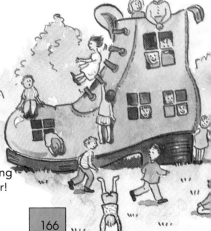

About 100 years ago, mothers quite often had more than ten babies. Sometimes all of them grew up to have children of their own, but usually some of them were too weak or small to live very long. People - especially mothers with a lot of children - were less healthy in those days, and doctors didn't know how to prevent weak babies from dying.

Nowadays, though, doctors can often save the lives of even the tiniest, weakest babies.

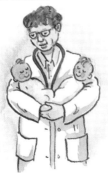

TOO MANY

WHAT IF EVERY WOMAN HAD AS MANY BABIES AS SHE COULD?

The most obvious thing which would happen is that families would be very, very big! But supposing every family had ten children, what would happen to the world?

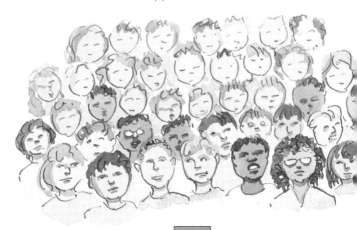

If every pair of parents made ten new people, the number of people in the world would become five times bigger. If there were two children for each two parents, then the population would stay the same.

In fact, the world's population has become more than twice as big since your parents were born (in about the last 50 years). Before your parents were born, it took nearly a hundred years for the world's population to double - and before that it took 150 years.

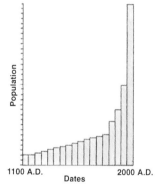

Before that, it took 600 years! Since the time of William the Conqueror, the number of people in the world has gone up ten times, from half a billion to five billion.

OVERLOAD

Because babies don't often die nowadays, and because people live to be much older, the number of people in the world is growing bigger and bigger, faster and faster. But the world doesn't get bigger, it stays the same size. This means everybody gets a smaller and smaller share, until one day there just won't be enough to go around. Some people think this has nearly happened already.

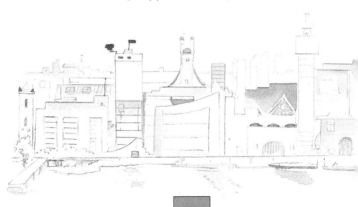

WHAT IS BIRTH CONTROL?

Birth control means not starting a baby until and unless we want to. It means that every baby that is born can have the best possible chance to be wanted and loved, in a home where there is enough room and enough to eat, and in a world where there's enough room, too.

The way we control how many babies we have, and when we have them, is called contraception.

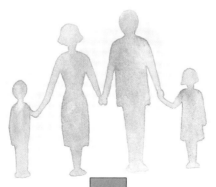

HOW DOES CONTRACEPTION WORK?

Contraception works by preventing an egg from being fertilised by a sperm. The simplest and most obvious way to do this is by putting a barrier in the way, something that will stop the egg and sperm meeting.

The two main kinds of barrier are the condom, also called sheath; and the diaphragm, also called a Dutch cap. A condom fits over a man's penis, and a diaphragm fits inside a woman's vagina to cover her cervix. Both are made of thin rubber.

Diaphragm

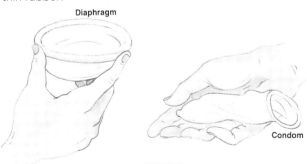

Condom

Another kind of barrier is a chemical one, which can be a cream or foam made of something which kills sperms, called a spermicide. Spermicide creams and foams are put into a woman's vagina before the man's penis enters. But spermicides alone do not work very well, so they are generally used at the same time as a rubber barrier.

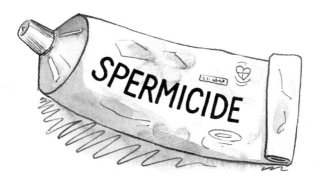

Condoms also prevent sexually-transmitted diseases (STDs) from passing between a man and a woman. A diaphragm does not protect either partner from catching these diseases.

Other types of contraceptives work in different ways, and no contraceptives except condoms also protect against disease.

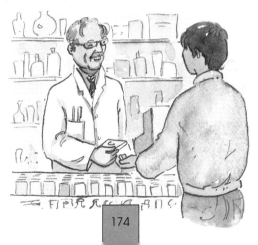

WHAT IS THE RIGHT WAY TO USE A CONDOM?

A new condom is packed all rolled up and ready to use. It must not be used if it has passed its sell-by date, or if it has been kept for a long time in a warm place.

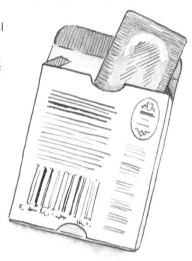

When using a new, fresh condom, it must be gently unrolled downwards to cover an erect (stiff) penis before the penis touches the partner's body. The small teat or bulb at the end should be pinched as the condom is fitted so that it stays loose, to leave room for the semen, but the rest of the sheath should fit closely all the way down.

Afterwards, it's important for a man to remove, or withdraw, his penis from a woman's vagina carefully, before it shrinks enough to allow any semen to escape. It is sensible to hold the condom in place while doing this. A condom is never used more than once; when it has been used it must be put into the toilet and flushed away.

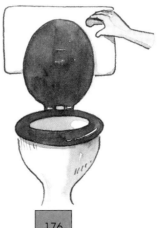

WHAT IS THE RIGHT WAY TO USE A DIAPHRAGM?

A diaphragm must be fitted by a doctor or nurse to make sure it is the right size. When a woman is fitted with a diaphragm, she will be shown how to use it. A diaphragm only works properly when it is used correctly by the person it belongs to.

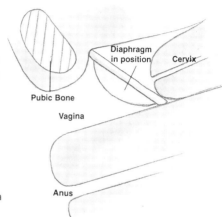

For extra protection, a woman can put some special cream (spermicide) or a tablet (pessary) inside her vagina before having sex using a condom or a diaphragm. This will help to destroy any sperms which may escape by accident.

177

WHAT IF SOMETHING GOES WRONG?

Very, very rarely, a condom can be damaged or split open while it is being used. If this happens, and a spermicide cream has not been used, it is a good idea to ask a doctor or the Family Planning Clinic for advice or help. In this case, it's best to visit the Clinic as soon as possible.

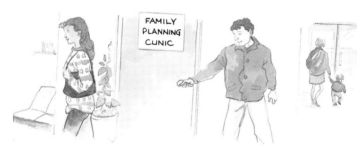

Diaphragms are made of thicker rubber than condoms, and if a diaphragm is cared for correctly it will last for a long time with no danger of damage.

WHAT IS THE PILL?

The Pill contains a small amount of sex hormone. There are many different kinds of contraceptive pill, but they all work by slightly changing a woman's hormones so that her ovaries and womb can't work together well enough to start a baby.

It is important to read the instructions carefully and always follow them properly. Because changing a person's hormones can have some effect on the rest of their body, taking contraceptive pills for a long time can make some women ill.

The morning after pill is sometimes used for emergencies, such as when a condom breaks. It can only be used with great care, and with the help of a doctor or the Family Planning Clinic, because the enormous amount of hormone it contains might make a woman feel very ill.

WHAT IS THE LOOP?

The loop, or coil, or IUD, is a specially shaped piece of plastic or wire which goes right inside a woman's womb. It has to be inserted by a doctor. Once the loop is in place, it stays there until the doctor takes it out again. Loops can cause problems for some women, though, and don't always prevent pregnancy.

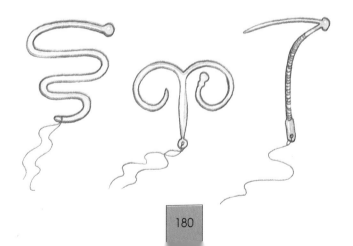

WHAT IS STERILISATION?

Married people who are quite sure they don't want to make any more new babies may decide to have a small operation to make certain that their eggs or their sperms can never meet the eggs or sperms of another person. For a man, this means sealing the sperm ducts so that sperms can't get into his semen. This is called a vasectomy. For a woman, it means sealing her tubes to make a barrier that eggs and sperms can't cross.

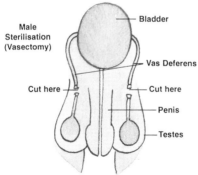

Male Sterilisation (Vasectomy)

Bladder

Vas Deferens

Cut here — Cut here

Penis

Testes

It may be impossible to reopen the tubes once they've been blocked, so a person must be quite certain he or she doesn't want any more babies before having this done. The operation is quick and simple for a man, but more difficult for a woman because her tubes are right inside her body. After this is done, it makes no difference to the way either men or women feel or the way their bodies work. A woman will continue having periods, and a man's penis will work normally.

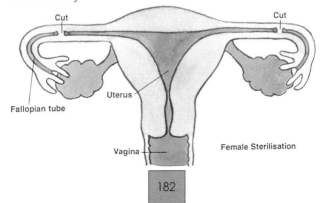

Cut

Cut

Fallopian tube

Uterus

Vagina

Female Sterilisation

WHAT IS THE RHYTHM METHOD?

The rhythm method (safe period) depends on two things. The first is that there are only a few days each month when an egg can be fertilised, and the second is that sperms can't survive for more than two days inside a woman's body.

Sun	Mon	Tue	Wed	Thu	Fri	Sat
	1	2	3	4	5	6
7	8	9	10	11	12	13
14	15	16	17	18	19	20
21	22	23	24	25	26	27
28	29	30	31			

183

So, if two people don't make love (have sex) for about five days in the middle of the menstrual cycle - two days before the egg is released (to allow time for sperms to die) and three days afterwards (to allow the egg to pass through the tube without meeting a sperm), this reduces the chance of starting a baby. But it depends on knowing (two days in advance!) exactly when an egg will be ripe.

This method of contraception is not suitable for women whose periods are not regular and, because it is even possible to start a baby while a woman is actually having her period, it is not a reliable method of contraception for any woman.

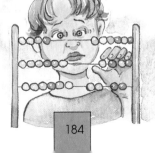

WHAT IS NOT A CONTRACEPTIVE?

There are some things that people believe which are simply not true.

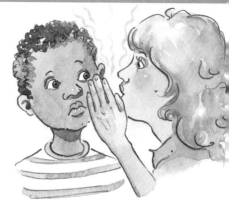

* It is not true that a woman or girl can't make a baby (become pregnant) the first time she has sex. Once she's started having periods (and even just before the first one happens), any girl can become pregnant if she has sex.
* It is not true that a man can withdraw his penis before he has a orgasm (ejaculates; climaxes; comes) to prevent a baby starting. Some sperms always leak out earlier than most of the rest, and only one sperm is needed to fertilise an egg.

* It is not true that a woman can't start a baby while she's having her period.
* It is not true that a woman can't become pregnant if she lies on top of a man or if they have sex standing up.
* It is not true that going to the lavatory, or rinsing out the vagina, or having a bath immediately after having sex will prevent a baby starting.

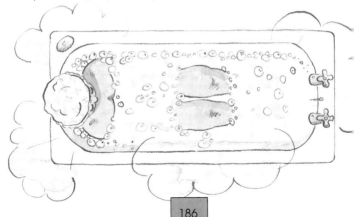

* It is not true that a woman can't become pregnant if she doesn't have an orgasm, or even if the man doesn't have an orgasm.
* It is not true that a woman can't become pregnant if she and her partner have sex in water.

The truth is that any direct contact between a man's unprotected penis and a woman's unprotected vagina, at any time, in any place or in any way, can start to make a baby.

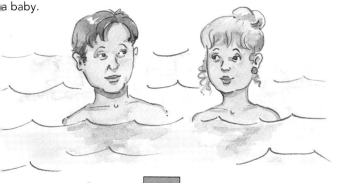

187

DICTIONARY

Here are the meanings of some more words which you might hear or see.

Adultery: sex between someone who is married and a person who is not their marriage partner

Anus: the opening where solid wastes come out

Arousal: sexual feelings; causing sexual feelings

Brothel: a place where prostitutes work

Castration: removing a male's testicles

Celibacy: choosing not to have sex

Change (the): see Menopause

Clap: a slang word for a sexually transmitted disease

Climax: ejaculation or orgasm

Copulation: the scientific word (for animals or people) for having sex (also mating or coitus)

Curse (the): a slang word for periods

Ejaculation: the moment when semen comes from a man's penis during sexual activity

Fantasies: unreal (imagined) things; sexual fantasies may be about doing things which aren't possible or allowed

Family planning: advice on contraception

Flasher: a person who inappropriately shows off their sex parts to strangers

French kissing: kissing which includes using tongues

Genitals: sex parts - penis, testicles, vagina, clitoris

Herpes: a kind of virus - one kind is an STD

Hysterectomy: an operation to remove a woman's womb

Lust: sexual desire, not necessarily through love, friendship or respect

Masochist: a person who enjoys being hurt

Menopause: the time when a woman stops having periods (about age 50), also called 'the change' or 'change of life'

Miscarriage: a pregnancy which ends naturally without a live baby being born

Necking: sexual cuddling and kissing

Nymphomania: an abnormal need (in a female) to have sex

Orgasm: ejaculation or sexual climax

Ovulation: the time when an egg leaves the ovary

Paedophile: an adult who sexually and illegally molests (interferes with) children

Perversion: abnormal (possibly illegal or forbidden) sexual behaviour

Petting: sexual touching

Platonic: non-sexual, usually meaning a type of friendship

Pornography ('porn'): writing, pictures, film or video made especially to arouse sexual feelings, often showing abnormal or otherwise unpleasant events

Premenstrual tension (PMT): feelings of discomfort and irritability in the few days before a woman's period starts, caused by hormone changes

Promiscuity: having sex with many people, without love ('sleeping around')

Prostitute: a person who has sex in exchange for money

Pubes: pubic hair

Sadist: a person who enjoys hurting others

Satyriasis: an abnormal need (in a man) to have sex

Smegma: stale skin and sweat which collects under the foreskin and must be cleaned away

Snogging: sexual cuddling and kissing

STD: sexually transmitted disease

Stillbirth: a baby which is born dead

DICTIONARY (cont'd) INDEX

Test-tube baby: a baby made by fertilising an egg with a sperm, outside a woman's body

Thrush: a common fungus disease sometimes affecting a woman's vulva

Titillation: causing sexual feelings (see also pornography)

Transvestite: a man who likes to wear women's clothes

Ultrasound: a safe way of seeing inside a person's body (without using x-rays); sometimes used to look at an unborn baby

VD (venereal disease): an old-fashioned name for an STD

Video nasty: an unnecessarily violent or pornographic film

Virgin: a person who has never had sex

Voyeur: a person who enjoys secretly watching other people doing private things (also called a 'peeping tom')

Whore: a slang word for prostitute